Autism Revealed

All you Need to Know about Autism, Autistic Children and Adults, How to Manage Autism, and More!

Table of Contents

Introduction iv

Chapter 1 - What is Autism? 1

Chapter 2 - Autism in Children............................... 7

Chapter 3 - A Parent's Guide 13

Chapter 4 - Autism in Adults 21

Chapter 5 - Autism and Aging............................. 27

Conclusion..30

Introduction

I want to thank you and congratulate you for downloading the book, *"Autism Revealed"*.

This book contains helpful information about Autism, and how it affects both children and adults!

If you are a parent of a child with autism, you will have a lot of questions. There are many challenges that you will face in the coming years, and how you handle your child's condition now may greatly affect them as they grow older.

This book explains what autism is, what may cause it, and its various signs and symptoms. No two cases of autism are the same, and therefore there are a variety of different treatment methods and techniques presented within this book.

This book will explain to you tips and techniques that will allow you to begin successfully understanding and managing autism. You will learn about how to manage autism at different stages of childhood, all the way up to adulthood.

Autism is a life-long condition. With the proper help and guidance, many autistic children grow up to live prosperous and somewhat normal lives. I hope this book is able to provide you with the knowledge and information required to make the correct choices for your child, and wish you the best of luck!

Thanks again for downloading this book, I hope you enjoy it!

Chapter 1 - What is Autism?

ASD or autism spectrum disorder is a range of complex neurodevelopment disorders. This medical condition has numerous symptoms including difficulties in communication, social impairments, and stereotypical, repetitive, and restricted patterns of behavior. Autistic disorder is also referred to as autism or classical ASD, and is considered the most severe form of ASD. The condition ASD also includes Asperger's syndrome.

This disability generally appears during the first three years of an affected person's life. It affects one's ability to communicate and interact socially. It is characterized by a set of behaviors and affects people differently.

Doctors often use the term *neurodiverse* for people afflicted with autism, as opposed to people who do not have the condition who are referred to as *neurotypical*.

Signs and Symptoms

ASD can produce a variety of signs and symptoms generally divided into two main groups. These are:

- Difficulty to communicate and interact socially. Issues include the impaired ability to understand other people's feelings and emotions. People who are suffering from autism often find it difficult to initiate conversations, or take part in any conversation for that matter.

- Repetitive and restricted patterns of physical behaviors, actions, thoughts, and interests. An autistic person is often seen making repetitive physical movements, like tapping their hand on the table. It upsets them if their routines are disrupted. Some even become violent when disrupted.

Common Signs and Symptoms

Spoken Language

- Delay in learning a few words or totally not being able to speak
- Repetition of phrases and set of words
- Monotonous to flat speech
- The preference to answer in single words even if the patient is capable of speaking in full sentences

Social Interaction

- Failure to respond when called by their first names
- Rejecting and failing to respond to cuddling initiated by their parents or guardian

- Having feelings of resentment when someone asks them to do something
- Having little interest to interact with other people, even kids their age
- Prefers to be alone rather than be around kids of the same age
- Not enjoying social gatherings, like birthday parties
- Avoiding eye contact

Behavior

- Doing repetitive movements, like flapping their hands or rocking back and forth on their seats
- Playing with a particular toy or toys in a repetitive manner. For instance, sorting out blocks and arranging them according to their colors in a straight line, as opposed to building something out of those building blocks.
- Prefers to follow a certain routine and tends to get upset when the routine is disrupted.
- Feeling and expressing a strong like or dislike to a particular food, based on taste or appearance.

According to experts, people diagnosed with ASD also usually have other mental conditions, like ADHD or attention deficit hyperactivity disorder, depression, or anxiety. Almost half of those people diagnosed with ASD have different levels of learning disabilities or difficulties. However, it is important to point out that with the right support, it is possible to help people with ASD to live independently. The support of not just their immediate family, but also the whole community and the society in general can make a huge difference in a person's life.

Causes of Autism

Researchers and doctors still haven't found the exact causes of ASD, but they have reason to believe that a variety of genetic and environmental factors could be involved. The causes can be categorized into two types:

Primary ASD (Idiopathic ASD) – There are no underlying factors that can be pinpointed as to how and why ASD developed.

Secondary ASD – Underlying medical conditions and environmental factors are said to put a person at high risk of developing ASD.

Risk Factors

- Genetic – Experts say that there are genetic mutations that may put a child at greater risk of developing ASD. Researchers believe that some genes inherited from the parents can make them more susceptible to developing autism. There have been reported cases of siblings having ASD, and it is not surprising to experts to find identical twins with the condition.

- Environment – The child in the mother's womb might have been exposed to some environmental factors that put them at risk of developing ASD. Most experts theorize that a person is born with a vulnerability to developing ASD, and the condition can further develop when a person is exposed to environmental triggers.

- Psychological – People who have been diagnosed with ASD may have certain thoughts that can contribute to further developing the symptoms. The *theory of the mind* concept is a person's ability to understand and recognize other people's mental states, while they themselves try to understand their own. Experts simply put it as "seeing the world through the eyes of another person".

- Neurological factors – There might be certain issues with the brain's development that may affect the nervous system and contribute to ASD symptoms. There are medical theories that suggest that ASD occurs when some parts of the brain, like the cerebral cortex, the limbic system, and the amygdala experience extreme emotion response to something trivial. This may also be the reason why autistics prefer routine movements in order to prevent triggering extreme emotional reactions to certain events or outside movements.

- Other medical conditions might also contribute to increasing the risk of certain individuals in developing ASD. Down's syndrome and cerebral palsy could be related.

The succeeding chapters will give you more information about child and adult autism and the different techniques the people around the sufferers can use to help them cope with this lifetime condition.

Chapter 2 - Autism in Children

Like every parent, you probably do not want to believe that your precious baby has a medical condition that has no cure. It is difficult, especially if it is ASD. However, doctors are one in saying that early detection, particularly within the first 18 months of the baby, could make a huge difference. However, no matter when autism was diagnosed, you, as a parent, should never lose hope because while there is no known direct cure, there are treatments that can effectively reduce the effects and let your kid grow in "normal" conditions.

Understanding Autism Spectrum Disorder

Autism is a spectrum of related medical conditions. It may appear during infancy or early childhood. Autism can cause holdups in the different areas of a child's development, like talking, playing, and interacting with other people.

Signs and symptoms differ. Some children with autism may only show mild impairments, while there are others who may have a number of challenges to cope with. Every child with autism often experiences problems in three basic areas. These are:

- Verbal and non-verbal communication
- Thinking and behaving

- Relating to the world around them

Watch Out for Early Signs and Symptoms

The child's parents are in the best position to catch early warning signs of ASD. Nobody knows your child better than you because you are the one who spends the most time with them. Your child's doctor can be an excellent partner in the early detection of this condition, but it is important to have your own observation and experience with your child.

Every parent needs to learn what is normal and what is not, in relation to autism.

- It is important that you monitor the development of your child. You have to observe closely if the general emotional, cognitive and social milestones of your child are achieved. However, a delay in development does not necessarily mean autism, but it can be a developing risk.

- There are kids who may develop ahead of others. It is normal. If you have had kids prior to a child in question, please note that every child develops at a different pace. If you suspect that something might be wrong, then take note of your observations and consult your child's pediatrician.

- Do not go the "wait-and-see" route. You might hear this from friends whom you might have consulted. However, for a parent, it is difficult to wait, especially if you suspect that something is amiss. Whether the main cause of the delay is autism or other factors, you do not want to lose any precious time for your child's proper development.

- As a parent, you should always trust your instincts. If you feel that something is wrong, do not delay in consulting your doctor or seeking a second opinion.

Babies and Toddlers

You should be looking out for these signs and symptoms:

- Your child does not make eye contact.
- Failure to respond when he/she hears your voice or when you are calling his/her name
- Does not smile back
- Does not make gestures to communicate
- Absence of making noises to gain attention
- Does not respond or even initiate cuddling
- Failure to copy your movements or facial expressions
- Failure to reach out when being picked up
- Does not show interest in the toys that he/she might be seeing around
- No spoken words (normally, a child can begin speaking his/her first word at 16 months)

For Older Children

There are red flags that you need to be on the lookout for in older children. As your child with autism gets older, the symptoms might elevate.

Basic Social Interaction

Children with autism have difficulty interacting socially. Most of these kids prefer to be left alone, they become detached, and aloof.

- They do not know how to interact with other people.
- They appear to be unaware or uninterested with what is going on around them.
- They do not like to be touched or held.
- They have trouble talking about their feelings to others, even to their parents.
- They appear to be disinterested or do not listen when another person talks to them.
- They do not play the "normal" games children play, like "pretend games". They also do not like playing with a group of kids.

Verbal Communication

- Most kids with autism learn how to talk later than normal.
- They often speak in an abnormal tone of voice. Most of the time, they speak in a certain pitch or rhythm.
- They repeat phrases and words non-stop.

- They respond to questions made by other people by repeating the question.
- They find it hard to communicate what they want.
- They often refer to themselves in the third person.
- They fail to follow simple instructions.

Non-Verbal Communication

- They avoid making eye contact.
- Their facial expressions often do not match what they are saying.
- They come off as robotic or unresponsive.
- They make limited hand gestures and movements.
- They can be sensitive to loud sounds.

Flexibility

- They follow a routine. However, any disruption to their usual routines can cause them to react violently.
- They have difficulty adapting to change.
- They often develop a strong attachment to something. It can be a toy, or key, or even light switches.
- They often show behaviors of being obsessively compulsive, like arranging things in a specific order that only they can understand.
- They can spend long periods of time doing a single activity, like arranging their things or focusing on a

certain part of an object, like the door or wheels of their toy car.
- They have repetitive movements.

The next chapter will give you detailed guidelines on how you can help your child cope with autism.

Chapter 3 - A Parent's Guide

Parents who have children with autism should not lose hope, for there are many things that they can do to help their kids overcome the challenges and obstacles they may face. However, as a parent, you have to realize that you cannot do it alone. You will need all the help you can get.

Taking care of a child with autism can take its toll on your own health. You need to be emotionally strong to be able to provide for, and understand the needs of, an autistic child. These tips can prove to be helpful in making your life and your autistic child's life easier.

Initial Reaction

If your child has just been diagnosed with ASD, then you may be wondering what lies ahead. No parent is ever prepared to learn that a child is anything but healthy. Not long ago, little information was known about autism. With advancements in technology and further studies, plus the growing awareness about the condition, it is no longer as challenging to cope with. Of course, autism can be frightening for a parent because it is never going away.

There is no cure for autism, but there are a number of ways to make your child's life easier. One cannot simply "grow out" of it, but you can help you child lead a normal life.

Important Tips to Remember

Learn About Autism

The more you know about the condition, the better equipped you will become to arrive at the right decisions when it comes to your child's well-being. Education is the key to finding ways to improve the life of your child.

Get to Know Your Child Better

Learn what triggers your child's tantrums or disruptive behaviors. Know what actions may illicit positive responses from him/her. Learn what calms him/her down. Know and understand what events or happenings affect them the most.

Accept your Child

It is never easy to accept the fact that your child is sick. Instead of focusing on your child having autism, shift your focus on what your child means to you. He/she may exhibit unusual behaviors, but he/she is still your child. Do not compare them with other children. If your child feels unconditional love and acceptance from his/her family, then they will feel it and appreciate it.

Do Not Give Up on your Child

No matter how difficult the road may be, you should never give up. Your child will need you to be strong and support them through the challenges they face.

How to Help your Child with Autism

Structure and Safety

- Consistency is important. Autistic children find it hard to adapt with the things taught to them in a single setting. For instance, your child might have learned to use sign language as a means of communication in school, but you fail to use it at home. Your child needs consistency to be able to continue the learning process. Encourage your child to apply at home what he/she has learned in school. You might also want to learn sign language so you can also use it to communicate with them at home.

- Follow a schedule. Autistic children can perform better if they follow a routine. This is still a part of being consistent. Set a daily schedule and strictly follow it. Set a schedule for meal times, school, therapy, and sleeping time. Try not to create disruptions or if there are any, limit them to a minimum. Should there be unavoidable changes, you need to make sure that you let the child know ahead of time.

- Give him/her a reward for every good behavior. Experts agree that it creates a positive effect on autistic children if people around them recognize them for doing something good. Acknowledge and praise your child even for the smallest achievements. A reward may be in the form of a favorite meal or even a smiley sticker. You do not need to be grand to be effective.

- Make your home child-friendly. It is important for an autistic child to have a space that he/she can call their own. Give them an area where they can feel secure and safe. You may put up labels or signs to define their "territory". However, it is important that you make the area safe, especially if your child is prone to tantrums or extreme behaviors.

The Power of Communication

Communicating with an autistic child is challenging. You need to communicate in order to understand each other. You do not necessarily need to talk just to communicate because there are a number of other ways to do so.

- Go for the non-verbal cues. It is important that you observe every action of your child. Look at his/her non-verbal actions. Most autistic children may find it hard to express themselves in words, but they can easily communicate through their actions and gestures. Pay attention to your child's facial expressions, to the sounds he/she makes, or to the hand movements and other gestures they makes when they wants something or are hungry.

- Learn what triggers their tantrums. It is a natural reaction for any child, autistic or not, to become upset and throw a tantrum. However, it is more difficult for a child with ASD since he/she may become violent. You have to identify the triggers because most of the time, a child with autism expresses their frustrations or disappointments through tantrums, for the simple reason that they do not know any other way.

- Find time for your child to have fun. Being a child should be fun. When you set a daily schedule, you have to make sure that there is a time for recreation. Play with your child. It is an essential part of the learning process.

- Do not neglect his/her sensory sensitivities. Most children with ASD are hypersensitive to sound, light, taste, smell, and touch. Others are "under-sensitive". You need to know what the sounds, movements, sights, or smells that trigger your child's disruptive behaviors are. You need to know what causes him/her to get stressed and what things can calm them down. Learn what activities are enjoyable for your child. Learn about the things that make them uncomfortable, too. It is important to learn these things so you can prevent them, know how to handle them when they arise, and give your child good experiences.

Create a Treatment Plan

While there is no direct cure, there are treatment options available. It may be hard to choose since every child is different. When you are deciding which treatment plans could be appropriate for your child, remember that you cannot find a single treatment that works for everyone. Since each child has his or her individual strengths and weaknesses, each would require different approaches.

To help you decide, keep in mind that a good treatment plan will:

- Help build your child's interests
- Offer a fixed schedule of activities
- Teach your child tasks that he/she needs to learn in a series of easy-to-follow steps
- Ensure to engage your child's attention with highly structured activities
- Involve the parents in the treatment

When you are looking for a treatment option, you have to identify your child's strengths and weaknesses. You also have to make sure that you know what behaviors are causing more problems. Make sure that you identify the skills that your child may be lacking. Know how your child is able to learn best, if it is through hands-on activities or simply watching or listening to instructions.

It is not enough to choose the most appropriate treatment plan. You have to make sure that you and your spouse involve yourselves in the treatment. You may also need the help of a good therapist.

The best way to choose the right treatment is to consult with your doctor and weigh in on all the options, with all the above factors in mind.

Finding Help and Support

It is not easy to care for a child with autism. You will need to devote your time and energy. There will be days when you will feel overwhelmed, discouraged and tired. It is hard enough to be a parent. It is even harder to care for a child with autism.

Considering all of these factors, you have to make sure that you also take care of yourself. Keep in mind that you do not have to do it on your own. You and your spouse can get a lot of help, aside from your family. One of the best ways is through support groups.

- Join support groups. You may find an autism support group in your area where you and your spouse can join. Families with autistic children often meet to share each other's experiences. You can learn from these people and get emotional support. It is easier to cope with the situation when you know that your family is not the only one having these problems.

- Look for a respite care center. You should also make sure that you stay healthy. Parents need a rest sometimes; otherwise, you will succumb to stress. A respite care center provides a caregiver who can temporarily take care of your child when you take a rest. It can be for a few hours, a few days, or weeks. You may ask your support group or your doctor for recommendations.

- Seek support from friends or even family counselors. It is inevitable that you will deal with extreme stress. It is also normal to feel depression at some point, especially when you have just recently found out about your child's condition. It is easy to feel overwhelmed. Therefore, you need support from your family and friends. You may also consult with a marriage or family counselor. You might also be comfortable in seeking advice from your local church priest or pastor.

Problems and challenges are normal in every household. What makes it more challenging is that you have to deal with an autistic family member. It is not just for the benefit of the parents, but also for the other children (if you have any), too. Some kids might not be able to understand what is going on with their sibling, and you might need the help of a professional to make sure that the other children understand the situation.

Chapter 4 - Autism in Adults

Autism is a lifetime medical condition. Doctors believe that if a child with autism is able to get the right treatment and support, he/she will grow up independently and assured of a good life despite having the medical condition. However, some people with autism grow up without a proper diagnosis. A diagnosis is imperative in giving the proper treatment and support; hence, parents really have a huge part in the early detection of the condition.

A child with autism transitioning into adulthood can be quite a challenge. For one, the child needs to transition from federally mandated services through the educational system to adult services. The public education privilege ends when the child turns two. However, the Individuals with Disabilities Education Act mandates that the transition should begin when the child turns 16. He/she will have to become a formal member of the IEP or Individualized Education Plan.

The transition is a lot of work, which is why your child needs your support and assistance along the way.

Diagnosis

Getting an accurate diagnosis for adult autism is quite hard. The symptoms could mean a number of medical conditions. Most doctors refer an individual to a clinical psychologist or psychiatrist for proper evaluation and diagnosis. Some of the vital areas to consider in adults with autism are the following:

Communication

- An adult with autism still finds it hard to decode gestures and body language of other people.

- It is still difficult to communicate with others.

- Not socially motivated because they do not know how to start or join a conversation.

- Not too many friends because of the failure to socialize.

Understanding

- An adult with autism finds it hard to be part of a group.

- Short conversations annoy them.

- They have trouble understanding conversation topics with double meanings and they tend to take things literally.

Thought Flexibility

- As adults, they are still fixated in pattern movements and routine activities.

- They have difficulty making future plans for themselves.

- They have trouble organizing even the simplest aspects of their lives.

- They still have trouble following directions.

- They encounter difficulty in coping with step-by-step tasks.

Getting a diagnosis for an adult with autism has several benefits. For one, it helps the individual to better understand themselves. It also helps rule out more serious mental problems, like schizophrenia. An accurate diagnosis can help you seek better treatment for your child as an adult.

What is Life Like?

People with autism exhibit common problems with social interaction and communication. These are the main causes of the challenges they have to face in life. An adult with ASD will have to be cared for by the family once he/she reaches the age of 21.

An adult with ASD will need a nurturing environment, not just in the home, but also at school and at work. It is still a learning process for the individual with ASD. Some adults with autism get employment and become successful in mainstream jobs. It might surprise you to know many autism sufferers grow up to become a success.

It may be necessary for your adult child to stay with you, but if you have provided the right treatment for them, it may not be as difficult as you envisage.

Some adults with autism are able to live independently. Some even live in their own house or semi-independently in their parents' house. They are provided with assistance when they need to solve major issues, and this can be from family, friends, or a professional agency.

For those who have opted to have the adult child with autism to live in their home, there are government funds available to help them. There are programs that include their own Social Security Disability Insurance or SSDI, Supplemental Security Income or SSI, and Medical waivers.

There are institutions that accept adults with autism. Most of those being sent here are those who need extensive assistance and supervision. There are higher-functioning adults with autism who are even employed in these institutions.

Understanding their Behaviors

Adults with autism have unusual behaviors. It could mean two things: they are trying to communicate, or it is their way of coping with a particular experience or situation. Knowing what causes these behaviors can be helpful.

Anxiety and Autism:

Adults with autism find it hard to deal with anxiety. Even individuals without the condition experience difficulty in dealing with anxiety. You can help an adult with autism understand where the anxiety is coming from so it is easier to deal with the intense emotion and its effects.

Some of the symptoms of anxiety include having trouble sleeping, difficulty focusing on an assigned task, losing patience easily, and constantly worrying. It is important to identify what is causing the anxiety.

Steps to Manage Anxiety

- Get the individual with autism to maintain a diary where he/she can write about particular situations and how the experience is making them feel. This will help the individual understand the cause of their anxiety and help him/her manage the emotion better.

- Teach him/her some relaxation techniques. An autistic individual often finds it hard to relax. It is helpful to learn what activities that they enjoy. You may ask him/her to do such activities in order to relax them.

- It helps to talk to your child about what they feel.

Communication and Interaction

You may still encounter challenges in communication. You just need to remember to get back to the most effective methods. If you have been with your child since he/she was young, you know by now how to communicate with them effectively. An adult with autism is no different from a child with autism.

If you can communicate with your child verbally and non-verbally, then it may not be as difficult. Essentially, if your child can easily communicate with the outside world as a child, he/she will not have difficulty when transitioning into adulthood.

Chapter 5 - Autism and Aging

Adults with autism can live a normal life, with proper support and treatment. What happens if they leave to live without their parents? How can you prepare your child to live without having you around?

Teach your child to learn to take care of his/her health, first and foremost.

One of the most important things an adult with autism has to do is to have lots of physical activities. An active lifestyle helps improve their health and well-being. If they go out often, then it is also easier to stay in touch with the local community, making it easier to ask for assistance if needed.

It is important to keep on learning and maintaining a high interest in life. Exercise can also help to manage stress.

Employment

Can an autistic adult find work? Yes, they can!

There are agencies that can assist adults with autism. Most individuals are able to finish school, thus making them eligible for employment.

There is a small percentage of adults with autism who are able to work in mainstream industries successfully. Individuals with autism can be highly skilled, and while some employers recognize that, there are still some who do not. There are institutions and agencies that can help an adult with autism find employment according to his or her educational attainment and skills.

There are three employment possibilities a person with autism has: competitive, supported, and secure/sheltered.

Competitive employment is for autistic adults who are highly independent. There are even highly skilled adults with autism who are able to manage their own businesses. Individuals with autism are likely to succeed in careers that need them to focus on details, but with limited interaction with his/her colleagues, like in computer programming and software development.

Supported employment supports individuals with autism to find paid employment within the community. They can find work as a mobile crew, or a position that is specifically tailor-made for the individual with autism.

Secure/sheltered employment guarantees an individual to be in a facility-based setting. In this kind of setting, the individual receives work skills and training.

Finding employment has never been easier than now with technology. An individual with autism can easily find many employment options. You can get a listing from the internet. There are agencies that offer assistance. It is just a matter of knowing where to get help and support.

Society in general is slowly getting educated on autism spectrum disorder, thus making the lives of those suffering from the medical condition easier.

Conclusion

Thank you again for downloading this book!

I hope this book was able to help you learn more about Autism!

The next step is to put this information to use, and begin better understanding and managing Autism!

Finally, if you enjoyed this book, please take the time to share your thoughts and post a review on Amazon. It'd be greatly appreciated!

Thank you and good luck!

www.ingramcontent.com/pod-product-compliance
Lightning Source LLC
LaVergne TN
LVHW021744060526
838200LV00052B/3454